Héctor Mario Lavalle

LEGAL ANSWERS TO COMMON MEDICAL QUESTIONS HABITUALS

Héctor Mario Lavalle

LEGAL ANSWERS TO COMMON MEDICAL QUESTIONS HABITUALS

Prevention of malpractice suits

ScienciaScripts

Cover image: www.ingimage.com

This book is a translation from the original published under ISBN 978-613-9-46694-8.

Publisher:
Sciencia Scripts
is a trademark of
Dodo Books Indian Ocean Ltd. and OmniScriptum S.R.L publishing group

120 High Road, East Finchley, London, N2 9ED, United Kingdom
Str. Armeneasca 28/1, office 1, Chisinau MD-2012, Republic of Moldova, Europe
Printed at: see last page
ISBN: 978-620-8-32842-9

LEGAL RESPONSES TO COMMON MEDICAL QUESTIONS. PREVENTION OF MALPRACTICE SUITS.

PRESENTATION

This paper was inspired by the concerns of doctors and lawyers themselves, the other party investigated by us, as we are convinced that knowledge is the best weapon for the prevention of lawsuits against the medical profession and health care teams.

The spirit is obviously legal, since doctors must always bear in mind that the person who will judge them will not be another colleague but a lawyer who will be the judge at the time, while bearing in mind that medical reasoning is not always consistent with legal reasoning.

Many answers were directly based on the guidelines of Law 17132, the new Civil Code and other legislation together with the Code of Ethics of the Argentine Medical Association in its third edition, the Code of the Argentine Medical Federation and our own contributions.

What is important is that by knowing the legal rules in advance the practitioner will know when his or her behaviour is lawful or unlawful, or can be challenged.

The idea is that knowledge decreases the daily stress of the professional and will lead you on the path to greater peace of mind in your daily activities.

In short, we don't want to prove anything, but simply to show and promote reflection.

CONTENTS

INTRODUCTION

Undoubtedly, the phenomena that occurred in the USA and Europe are quickly replicated in the peripheral countries, so that medical liability lawsuits do not originate in South America.

The uncontrolled increase has had a double effect. First of all, a primary defence mechanism on the part of the medical profession, which, among other things, took refuge in what is known as defensive medicine, spending an incalculable amount of money in both the private and state spheres, without at least achieving a higher quality of medicine.

Secondly, it is a terrible attack on the greatest asset a professional can have, which is his reputation, his prestige and, why not, his honour.

There are multiple factors that generated this out-of-control increase in legal claims by patients, among which we can cite a population that underwent Copernican changes undreamt of since the middle of the 20th century and as a first consequence no longer felt like a patient, but rather a consumer and claims from that position as such.

Accompanied by the extinction of the family doctor who for years cared for the whole family and who was replaced by an institutional and impersonal medicine.

In Argentina, the second national sport seems to be doctor hunting.
and some hunters have been able to land important game.

This situation leads the professional to a state of fear that makes his or her work and well-being feel threatened by uneasiness rather than joy for such a noble profession.

This is not to deny the medical malpractice that undoubtedly exists in many cases. So far it seems that the best way to fight this real scourge is prevention through knowledge, which we will try to do by answering questions we hear from colleagues themselves. In addition to what has been said above, we believe that a deficient communication system on the part of the medical staff, not only to the patient but also to the patient's relatives, must also be added to the genesis of these problems.

To inform is not to communicate.

MEDICAL LIABILITY AND THE NEW CIVIL AND COMMERCIAL CODE

1- What did the new Civil and Commercial Code substantially change in terms of the What does it mean for doctors in their daily work?

Emphasises the preventive function.

Avoiding unjustified damage and not aggravating it if it has already occurred Art 1708 In terms of compensation: it unified the contractual and extra-contractual orbit.

The full reparation of the damage is enshrined, which includes not only the compensatory capital, but also loss of earnings and medical expenses, the corresponding interest and the costs of the process that the creditor has been obliged to pay for the initiation of the trial. It seems to us necessary to point out that doctors treat patients and it is only fair to differentiate between the harm caused by the alleged medical damage and the harm caused by the illness itself that led to the consultation,

It also deals with non-pecuniary damage, formerly non-pecuniary damage, which gives it a very broad meaning.

Gives children and young people more decision-making power

The aforementioned 13-16 year olds have the capacity to decide on non-invasive medical treatments and not on particularly risky ones.

The parents shall attend when the treatment presents these conditions. Art.26.

From the age of 16, an adult is considered to be an adult for care decisions.
of his body.

It should be noted that it is not easy to determine what is aggressive and what is not aggressive and that there can be enormous differences between 13 and 16 years of age, not only physical but also in terms of maturity, psychic etc., which requires greater attention on the part of the professional.

For adults

The principles of autonomy and presumption of competence are in force. Competence decision-making. It emphasises personal rights and the autonomy of will, i.e. dignity, which involves the rights to integrity and life. These anticipated rights correspond to Art. 60.

These are decisions that involve or reject treatments that carry risks.

2- What does Art. 60 specifically say? It pertains to advance medical directives
The fully capable person can anticipate directives and confer a mandate in respect of his or her health in anticipation of his or her own incapacity.

It may also designate the person or persons who are to express consent to medical acts and to exercise guardianship.

Directives involving euthanasic practices are considered to be unwritten

3- How are these directives implemented?

It must be formalised in writing before a notary public or a court of law.
First Instance with two witnesses.

4- Does it have to go through the same process to revoke this mandate?

It can be revoked orally, with the presence of two witnesses and their signatures.
in the medical record together with that of the treating physician.

Does the unification of contractual and non-contractual liability reduce the limitation period?

Under the previous Code the patient had the time limit of ten years to sue in the contractual relationship, which applies to almost all medical liability suits. In tort 2 years. In the current Code, the time for the patient is reduced to three (3) years, since whether in the contractual or non-contractual relationship.

Thus, if more than three years have passed, the claim of the patient. Again, in the previous Code it was 10 years.

Informed consent

5- Is informed consent always an obligation?

It is an obligation unless otherwise stipulated, and is an exception in cases of emergency where life-threatening or seriously incapacitating circumstances may occur or where no qualified persons are available.

Informed consent is mandatory in cases which are not surgery?

No one may be subjected to clinical or surgical examinations or treatment without their free and informed consent unless otherwise provided by law. Art 59 Civil Code.

Without prejudice to special provisions, the free and informed consent of the injured party, in so far as it does not constitute an unfair term, releases him from liability for consequential damage. This is stated in Art. 1720.

What is not in the consent is evidence to the contrary.

6- If the patient is not in a position to give it, who can do it for him or her?

The legal representative, the spouse, the partner, the cohabitant, the relative, the one who accompanying or related.

Organ transplantation

7- Is organ procurement allowed in Argentina?

The human body has no commercial value for our Code but has affective, therapeutic, scientific, humanitarian or social value and can only be made available if some of these values are respected and as provided for by special laws (art. 17), i.e. they are non-patrimonial goods.

8- What if contracts are signed that specify a commercial value? Contracts with such a purpose are null and void.

People with disabilities.

The law presumes their capacity, the idea being to ensure and guarantee the greatest possible degree of autonomy, but which admits the application of exceptional limitations that benefit the disabled person.

9- Can people with limitations make decisions about their health?

The Code presumes them competent to receive information and make decisions about their health, confirming the principles of progressive autonomy and presumption of competence.

10- When is a health professional not liable for an act of a health professional? unlawful?

When a state of necessity arises or when there is consent without justification. An example is triage in the case of disasters.

11- What is the meaning of unlawfulness?

Any act or omission that causes harm to another is unlawful -art 1717.

In the contractual sphere a type of typical unlawfulness persists where the damage is the consequence of the breach of a specific obligation, whether arising from a contract or not.

Reparation of damages.

12- What is the scope?

Immediate and foreseeable damage must be compensated (art. 1726).

That is to say, those that tend to happen according to the natural course of events and ordinary course of things.

Release of liability

13- Are there any factors that remove a physician's liability? The most common factors that interrupt medical liability are:

a- Non-compliance of the patient with medical instructions as well as the interruption of the treatment. Art 1729.

b- The act of a third party for which no liability is due that meets the conditions of an act of God. Art 1731

E.g. When a sanatorium is held responsible for an act for which it is liable another institution.

c- The limitations of science constitute an assumption of major cause.

MEDICAL GUILT

14- Is there a special guilt for doctors?

There is no such thing as medical fault, but it is governed by ordinary fault.

It should be noted that for most judges fault is of a subjective nature, so that the defendant's ault must be proven in order to assign subsequent attribution.

15- Some guidelines for assessing medical fault

1- Failure of medical treatment does not necessarily mean a failure to act.
professional negligence

2- The doctor cannot undertake to cure the disease, but only to put the patient at the centre of the disease.
The patient's service to the patient with all his science and diligence in the care of the patient.

3- The physician's fault begins when the scientific discussions end, for if there are several techniques and treatments for a case and the physician chooses one of them, there can be no claim that he or she might have prevented a death in the other way.

4- The professional's conduct must be assessed on the basis of the circumstances existing at the time of the challenged practice.

It is not the same to operate on peritonitis in a sanatorium or central hospital as it is to operate in a remote rural area with precarious equipment.

5-Correct treatment can lead to progress or regression of the disease. For this reason, changes in the patient do not necessarily mean or imply negligence on the part of the physician.

16- Irrespective of the Code and the opinion of the experts, what is the judges' view and what do they consider to be the parameters for measuring medical malpractice?

What they call the **standard of care** is the key that allows the judge to enter into the matter.

When medical conduct is not acceptable for a standard practitioner and his or her actions clearly fall below the standard of care, these are parameters that the judge has as a valid reference for judging.

The standard of care is not compared to optimal care but rather to care that
corresponds to the level of a reasonably prudent ordinary doctor.

Medical experts will give the judge an idea of the level of standard of care for the case in question.

This is the basis from which it will take medico-legal issues to move forward.

17- What is required for a judge to find a doctor guilty?

In the first instance, the judge will take legal concepts with a magnifying glass
medical focus.

For judges in our country, in order for liability to exist, there must be fault, **i.e. there is no liability without fault.**

We will then see which are the elements that the judge uses to study whether or not there was guilt or not.

First element:

There must actually be damage. Without which there is no basis for a claim.

It is when a right or interest that is not reprobated by the legal system and whose object is the person, the patrimony or a right of collective incidence is injured (art 1737 CC and CN).

The new Civil Code also enshrines **full compensation for damages** as a general principle (art. 1740 CC. and CN), which includes, in addition to the compensation capital, other concepts such as loss of earnings, medical expenses and the corresponding interest calculated from the time each damage occurs (art. 1748 CC. and CN).

Second element

The judge will see whether an infringement or violation of a **pre-existing legal duty** has been committed, e.g. what is expressly prohibited by ordinary laws, ordinances, regulations etc.

Not only for violation of the law, it is not limited to this concept alone, but extends to **not harming others**.

In law this second step is known as Antijuridicality. Third element
Establish authorship.

That is to say, if the harmful event for which the claim is made **can be attributed** by action or omission on the part of the defendant physician(s).

For fault to exist and for the professional to be considered as **the author of** the damage, it is indispensable that there must be a link between the medical action or omission and the damage caused, so that the damage can be legally imputed to the defendant.

In law it is known as **causal relationship**

Fourth element

Attribution factors

Formerly called imputability, which is nothing more than the concurrence of some subjective or objective factor that the law considers apt or suitable for one or more subjects to be liable.

As liability is a personal fact, the attribution factor is subjective, so that **by his actions he is the author of the damage and can be held at fault.**

Without compliance with these factors there will be no guilt.

18- Can unlawfulness be defined?

It is any action or omission that results in harm to another, in the absence of justification. Pursuant to art. 1717 of the new Civil Code.

When it violates the agreement, but also if it violates the provisions of a norm or **in the face of the general duty not to harm**.

But there are cases in which there is no medical liability, e.g. state of necessity (art 1718 CC and CN) as well as the consent of the injured party.

There are also grounds for justification if it is a matter of avoiding an otherwise unavoidable evil, and the triage performed by doctors in the event of a catastrophe is a good example of this.

DUTIES OF THE DOCTOR

19- What kind of obligation does the physician have to the patient?

Almost all of the duties of physicians are **of means.**

20- What is an obligation of means?

It consists of applying all the **care** and **diligence** required by their intervention in the performance of their professional task, taking into account the circumstances of the people, time and place. That is to say, in a way, also to comply with the scientific regulations for the case.

It imposes only diligence with measures that normally lead to an outcome or cure, **but no assurance that it will occur.**

In any case, we can say that conceptually medicine is care and, if possible, cure. A small number of medical acts correspond to an obligation **of results**, and that failure to achieve them begins the liability for not fulfilling the promised obligation.

These are acts like a transfusion... For example, reading and reporting a haematocrit. It is also to ensure a result...-

They are the fewest, as medical acts generally respond to **a responsibility of means.**

In the event of a breach of the obligations of means, this always entails
subjective liability. Proof of fault is **required** here.

In the case of a breach of an obligation of result, liability is strict, i.e. **it is not necessary to** prove medical fault, the effective conduct is assessed, the promised...

Proving that the expected performance was not fulfilled is sufficient, it is not necessary to prove fault. This creates a presumption of fault on the part of the debtor, i.e. the professional.

Fault is not necessary, diligence is not taken into account.

Only an act of God can exempt it from liability, and we reiterate that there is no liability without fault.

For civil liability to exist, there must be fault, damage and a causal relationship. Bueres quotes André Tunc who already stated this in 1981.

21- What do the judgements say about the obligation in cosmetic surgery?

It is specifically **an obligation of means**, which is supported by abundant jurisprudence, although the idea that it is an obligation of result still persists in some judges, who maintain that if they are not assured of a result, patients would not be operated on.

It is means-tested because the results depend on the alternatives of the patient that are beyond the scope of the technique used.

In medicine, even the simplest operation cannot guarantee a result, because medicine is the opposite of mathematics - unforeseeable risks can arise.

But let it be clear that the informed consent should include all possible alternatives.

In plastic surgery, it should not be understood that the physician is obliged to achieve the result sought by him and his client, but rather to diligently execute what science, technique and the medical art indicate as conducive to it, according to the circumstances of the people, time and place... (CNCiv. Sala I, 30/31990, PDC v. Morrone, Roque, LL, 1991-A-142).

In this speciality, whether restorative or cosmetic surgery is carried out on the Informed consent is in many cases at the heart of the matter.

The physician should not promise an outcome, but should disclose all reasonable possibilities of apparent non-compliance, so that any alternatives were already disclosed and accepted in the consent.

On the other hand, Law 17.132, which regulates the practice of medicine, prohibits in its Art.20 to advertise or **promise to** cure or preserve health.

So following that thought you cannot promise or assure a nose or cheekbones resembling an ideal that the patient has as a goal in her mind, but you must act as diligently as possible and follow the rules of lex artis.

The Codes of Ethics also prohibit practitioners of the healing arts from promises to secure an outcome.

But it must be borne in mind that there are still judges who are convinced that cosmetic surgery is an obligation of result, which makes doctors see justice as detached from reality.

Doctors' doubts about the suitability of some magistrates also increase when they read that a judge with years of experience in the judiciary was encouraged to write that in normal childbirth there is an obligation of result, since normal childbirth cannot generate risks that cannot be foreseen and controlled, as we will see in the conclusions.

Some judges, although they were counted on the fingers of one hand, adhered to this thinking, forgetting that in addition to the risks inherent in any birth, anaesthesia, blood transfusions, medicines, sutures, etc. can also be added.

Doctors do practical work as students and when they study different specialties they also study forensic medicine, it would not be idle if some of the many medical organisations in our country and in the world invited some judges to spend a day in a maternity ward and attend a maternity ward. with their presence in the delivery room to encounter the reality and the risks.

Surely some would appreciate the invitation, not to learn obstetrics but to get a general idea of what they have in their hands and what normal means in medicine. Generally one only talks about what one knows. The reasons are overwhelming for considering that obstetricians develop an obligation of means and not of result.

22- How long do patients have to file a lawsuit?

The new Civil Code unified the time when it comes to relationships
contractual and non-contractual.

Except for legal alternatives, we reiterate because of their importance, the time available to patients to sue **is three years.**

Ten years, as indicated in the previous Code in contractual relations, which are almost all of them, was unmerciful, as it kept the professional for ten years or more in a very prolonged anguish.

In other words, it unified the contractual and non-contractual relationship in three years.
In the previous Code, the non-contractual period was two years.

Type of doctor-patient relationship

Contractual:

It corresponds to a free agreement of wills between the physician and the patient, which, when it exists, generates a special type of contract that does not require any formalism and begins with the fact of medical care.

Non-contractual:

It arises from wrongful acts, whether intentional or negligent.

E.g., if a doctor is involved in the event of a traffic accident and attends to the injured, the relationship is also non-contractual.

23- What must be taken into account for a medical record to be constructed?
correctly and be assessed by the judge?

1- If it is done manually, it is essential for it to be legible and not to be modified at a later date, encrypted ...personal entry is essential for it to be valid.

2- **Again, most medical practices are in a contractual relationship**.

Society and the doctor

24- The fact that malpractice lawsuits are increasing exponentially
can this be interpreted as a significant decrease in the level of
professional responsibility?

Although there are main and accessory causes that generate judicial recourse on the part of patients, we can say that, broadly speaking, lawsuits are generated by multi-causal issues.

Lack of accountability as a general idea is a phenomenon that cannot be addressed by the
can hold it responsible for this excessive increase in litigation.

But we must look at this problem in the context of our society.

We can see on an almost daily basis truly incompatible facts that emanate almost always from the same sectors and that are visible to those who want to see them and that directly affect responsible behaviour.

The actors, as always, are the usual familiar faces. Any Argentine citizen, if questioned and with his or her mental faculties unscathed, as to which are the most irresponsible sectors in Argentina will surely tell you which ones with little margin for error.

One would have to be very basic to generalise, which is not the intention, as we know that there are exemplary and honourable sectors and even **martyrs** alongside other execrable ones.

Doctors are not born by spontaneous generation, they are in a way children of this society and as such they grow, develop and fortunately, only a few take some of their faults and forget their masters, which is also true for lawyers.

Is it a general problem? We do not know what the repercussions on society are, but exemplary behaviour is not abundant. In our society **there are** also **heroes** and victims among doctors and lawyers who are children of this heroism, and they are not few in number. The pandemic and **other acts** of courage and **death** in the justice system have demonstrated this.

However, there are problems in our society that are difficult to solve, such as the destruction of the principle of authority, which is not seen as a problem. only in the area of delinquency but also at school, in the family, in the workshop, in the street, etc. and the habituation or almost chronicity of a part of the population to live on handouts without working, giving no value to effort.

In this regard, the master physician Agrest wrote: / the physician must understand that his patients emerge in large numbers from this special, mediatic and sometimes incomprehensible kind of society, so that there is a very short step between this special kind of society from which patients emerge and a judicial claim......

25- Percentage of physicians in demand in the USA

In the US, 40% of general practitioners have a chance of being prosecuted once in their career. Some specialists have higher averages (American Medical Association). A.Dodge in Good Doctors Get Sued tells us that 25% of practicing physicians are prosecuted each year and that 50-65% of all physicians may be prosecuted during their careers.

26- How long does a doctor have to wait until the end of the trial in Argentina?

Approximately three to five years may be an average without counting the court time in case of an appeal.

Doctor-patient relationship

27- What is the importance of the doctor-patient relationship?

No one doubts that a good relationship is the best shock absorber and trial preventer. But current events call this kind of bond into question, as it passes insensitively from patient to consumer. As long as everything is within what the patient considers normal, everything is fine, but as soon as any unpleasant alternative happens, this pre-existing relationship vanishes within a few minutes.

In other words, whatever the cause of a complication, the doctor-patient relationship becomes a chimera; moreover, patients turn to institutions rather than to the doctor, and sometimes do not always know his or her name.

Given these circumstances, the physician should consider changing the name of the patient for **consumer.** Lawyers call it the client. It is the patient as a consumer of any product and when he considers that something is faulty he complains.

Exceptions exist and there are many of them. 29- What are dynamic loads? Again, in law, he who can prove wins.

In medical liability lawsuits, it is the **patient** who has to bear the burden of proving medical malpractice, a difficult task for obvious reasons. When the evidence is difficult, the judge can now resort to a reversal of the burden of proof, i.e. requesting the evidence from the person who is best placed to provide it, which in these cases is the doctors, while allowing them to make their own defence. It is a way of collaborating to find the truth of what happened, which the new Code authorises.

30- Liability of the private clinic

Summarising the theories on the subject, it is correct to think that when the clinic is not efficient in its work, either because of staffing failures or the things it uses, it is responsible.

ADVERTISING AND OFFERING OF SERVICES

31- Advertising behaviour.

Art. 79 of the Code of Medical Ethics of the Argentine Republic approved by COMRA states that the size and typeface of advertisements should be discreet.

Art. 80 of the Code of Ethics details which are the advertising behaviours that are against ethics and Art. 2 of Law 17.132, which determines advertising behaviours forbidden to health professionals.

The Code of Ethics. Art. 80

They are expressly against ethics:

a- Oversized advertisements with eye-catching characters or accompanied by photographs.

b- Those who offer the prompt, fixed-term and infallible healing of certain diseases

c- Those that promise free services or those that explicitly state o implicitly mention fee rates.

d- Only professionals who belong to the teaching staff of the university may advertise with the title of professor, provided that the professorship or subject of designation as such is specified.

e- Those transmitted by radiotelephony or loudspeakers, those made on cinematographic screens, those distributed in the form of flyers or cards which are not distributed b y post and to a specific addressee.

f- Signs or illuminated signs

g- Publicise thank you letters from patients.

As a general rule, advertisements should be sensible, moderate and prudent, i.e. as modest as possible.

Art. 20 of Law 17132 prohibits

1. Announcing or promising a cure by setting a time limit.

The doctor cannot guarantee the success of a treatment, but only the (CNCiv, Chamber E, 19/12/77.

They may require reasonable efforts to cure, but not promise to do so in the long term. beforehand (Resp.ED.1981-587)

32- Promise relief or cure by means of secret or mysterious procedures, as treatments must be those endorsed by the scientific community.

3 Publish false therapeutic successes, fictitious statistics, inaccurate data or any other deception.4...

33- What are the minimum standards for the licensing of a practice?

--Waiting room with direct access from the outside or common access in the case of horizontal property, with non-transparent doors and walls, which may be common to more than one consulting room and/or office and both at the same time if the activity is carried out by collaborators who have authorised private practice.

--The area of the waiting room shall be not less than nine metres.
squares.

--It shall have direct communication with the waiting room or transit areas where it is located, with non-transparent doors and walls and separated from the waiting room by a complete wall or partition, with no space between the ceiling and the waiting room.

--The surface area of the consulting room and/or cabinet shall be not less than seven and a half square metres, with adequate ventilation and air renewal systems.

DOCUMENTATION MEDICAL

34- What are the conditions that a medical certificate must meet? First of all, **veracity**.
It is an essential element and puts the signatory in a delicate situation if this condition is not met.

There are countless abuses so the time is not far off when the recipients of these certificates will decide to put an end to this practice of certificates when they are dubious....

Truthfulness can be violated with a proxy certificate or with a paid certificate, as there may be professionals who charge a fee for this.

Secondly, be as realistic as possible and avoid **exaggeration or magnification** if any ailment exists.

Thirdly**, it must be legible.**

It can be observed that medical writings are generally illegible, which marks a lack of consideration and contempt for those who have to read them, whether they are colleagues or not.

Perhaps someone might think that it is synonymous with academic prestige to writing in illegible form.

35- Is there a law that says what conditions must be met for a person to have a medical certificate?

Decree 6216/67, which regulates Law 17.732, stipulates that all the certificates shall be issued in:

a- Pre-printed forms containing

- Name and surname-date-signature-stamp
- Registration number
- Address

36- What are the consequences for a doctor of issuing a certificate false?

In principle, it constitutes a crime against public faith, and is contemplated in Article 295 of the Argentine Criminal Code.

Any doctor who gives a false certificate in writing concerning the existence or non-existence, present or past, of any illness or injury, when this results in harm, shall be sentenced to imprisonment for a period of one month to one year.

The penalty shall be from one to four years, if the false certificate results in a healthy person being detained in an insane asylum, lazaretto or hospital.

Even if the internment does not take place, the offence is consummated by the extension of the Certificate Is the recipient of a false certificate liable?

Injury, which may be of any kind, may be inflicted on a person to whom the false certificate has been issued or to a third party.

Article 296 of the Criminal Code imposes the same penalty as for the perpetrator of falsehood whoever makes use of a false or falsified document or certificate.

If the issuer of a false certificate is a public official, he shall be subject to the accessory penalty of absolute disqualification for twice the length of the sentence.

37- What is required for the medical record to serve as evidence?

Firstly, it must be reliable for the judge, i.e. it must not be subject to modification or different types of alteration.

For this purpose, it should be handwritten or with computerised medical records that ensure the inalterability, security, authenticity and chronology of the facts.

It must have an access code by means of a magnetised card, cryptography, biometric based methods, digital signature with date and time...

Cryptography is a mathematical process that converts information into a cipher text and requires a password to operate.

It should be noted that not all institutions are in a position to offer this information technology for access to medical records.

On an ordinary computer, anyone can log on and change or alter the text, so it is not evidence. Law 26529 in its art. 13 gives clear guidelines on computerised medical records: the content of the medical record can be made on magnetic support, as long as all the means are used to ensure that preservation, integrity, authenticity, unalterability, durability, durability and retrievability of the data contained therein in a timely manner. To this end, the use of restricted access with identification keys, control of field modifications or any other suitable technique to ensure its integrity should be adopted. The regulation stipulates that supporting documentation must be kept, and designates the persons responsible for the safekeeping of the documentation as being in charge of keeping all the sheets of paper.

3- Each sheet should have **the** patient's **name** on it

4- That no **blanks** are left

5- **Do not cross out** or amend. Error is put and signed,

6- **Date and time** of each medical care - **Date and time of** each medical care - **Date and time of** each medical care - **Date and time of** each medical care

7- That **inter-consultations** are listed in the same detail - that the same details are given

8- To be built **contemporaneously** with the facts

9- To be signed by the **acting** surgeon **or physician** and not by his assistant.

10- To be informed on what date and time the incumbent doctor is replaced. By e.g. holidays, travel etc.

11- **Telephone**, **internet** or other means of **consultation** should be recorded.

12- The patient's **non-compliance** must be recorded.

13- Details of the patient's condition **on admission** to the sanatorium or hospital such as also from the office consultation.

14- It should be supplemented by nursing charts.

15- If the diagnosis is not known, demonstrate that it is being pursued concretely.

16- The information to family members must be dated.

17- It must not contain **acronyms or abbreviations.**

Acronyms or abbreviations together with illegibility are two conditions that greatly irritate those who have to read the medical record, including the judge and some doctors as well.

19- Phrases such as s/p, compatible with, vital signs good, would appear to be, could be... good general condition... should not be used without explaining the meaning of each of these concepts in detail.

20- It must have incorporated the studies carried out.

21- All details of the transfer must be recorded.

An incomplete or flawed medical record does not in itself mean that malpractice has occurred, but it can be taken by the judge as a presumption against malpractice.

Often the medical history was used by the judge to take a decision on a case.
decisions against or in favour of the professional,

Unnecessary risk

38- Is there any risk in transcribing prescriptions generated at some point in time by another colleague or at the request of the applicant?

The risk is enormous and we will give the rationale.

1- You have signed a prescription without checking the patient.
2- You do not know your medical history
3- The colleague may have made a mistake, and you repeat the mistake.
4- Was the indicated medication correct 1 year ago? Is it correct at the time of transcribing the medication?
5- At the time of the transcription, you may be taking medication that alters the expected outcome and that you were not taking at the time of the first prescription.
6- The pharmacist may make a mistake and dispense another medicine.
7- The medication you are repeating may be in a poor condition of conservation
8- The route of entry into the body can be confused.

9- He does not know if it is appropriate at that time of the disease.

10- You do not know the actual disease at the time of repeating the prescription.

11. The requester can be wrong.

12- He is unlikely to show the original recipe, as he either brings the empty container or the name written on a piece of paper or he dictates it to himself as he knows it by heart.

13- The time when the first prescription was generated is unknown.

14. Themedication can aggravate pathologies pre-existing pathologies that previously did not exist.
15- Undecipherable lettering that causes the pharmacist to make mistakes and dispenses another medicine of a more or less similar name.

16- Self-medication is a widespread practice in our country.
half

The number of deaths due to medication errors that can be found in any manual together with the number of hospitalisations in routine practice shows us the risk also of routine and blind prescriptions and errors.

We don't know if this is possible in other latitudes, but in Argentina it is
a practice that still exists.

Judges bear in mind that medication is the final part of a process of examination, testing and diagnosis of the patient to be finalised if necessary with a prescription.

You do none of this when you transcribe a recipe.

Advance directives

39- What advance directives are provided for in the new Civil and Commercial Code?

It is a declaration of will made by an individual to have his will respected when he is deprived of his capacity for any reason.

40- If it does so in writing and at a given moment revokes its decision
orally, which decision must be respected by the physician.

The verbal revocation decision is valid and the physician must respect it.

Law 26529 provides for the possibility of revoking advance directives at any time.

41- Mechanism for giving effect to oral revocation

Two witnesses and the signature of the professional.

As far as documentation in general is concerned, it is not a question of accumulating documentation, but rather that it should be of good quality.

Quantity, if it is not of quality, helps very little.

The fact of accumulating documentation, in itself, is not a fact that frees the professional from responsibility.

For example, a 20-page medical record is of no use if it is poorly constructed or if the essentials are not well reflected.

Therefore, we can be sure that more does not mean better.

What is the use of a 30-page medical record if it is not well and thoroughly developed, e.g. what is the condition of the patient entering the sanatorium or hospital?

Or if the information is poorly organised and the judge finds it difficult to follow the sequence.

In summary, as Saxony Leaman says, the triad of documentation is: Comprehensive
Clear Concise

INFORMATION TO PATIENT

42- Information to patients and their relatives about the existing pathology and its evolution.

It is a universally accepted truth that the patient must know the reality of his or her disease, as well as its future and treatment.

Immediate family members must also know with the patient's consent, but cannot decide for the patient, if the patient's mental faculties are intact.

43- What should be taken into account in patient information when
have a terminal illness?

In principle, tell the truth, but taking into account some aspects to be considered, such as age, cultural and religious levels and the patient's knowledge in order to foresee negative reactions to information that implies a complicated and inexorable end.

Mystery, taboo and dissimulation aside, but with a component of piety.

Who would like to hear your doctor tell you that you have approximately three months to live? Or that you will have to be intubated and put on a ventilator without knowing how long it will last?

They harassed doctors so much with lawsuits that many rightly choose to copy the American model, i.e. the raw and hard truth to avoid problems, they put the doctor in these cases in front of the law and some comply with it to the letter.

The question is, who benefits from ruthless behaviour?

44- What is the medical conduct when the patient asks you not to want to
know anything, do what you have to do and don't report it?

In such cases, it must be ensured that the behaviour is real and does not represent a transitory issue.

If it is real, the patient's feelings must be obeyed and the next of kin must be informed of the case.

It is advisable to record this in detail in the medical record.

But it is important to keep in mind that there are patients who want to know about the truth, however hard it may be, and the doctor in such cases should consider that it is not only a question of telling the truth but also of **how the truth is told**.

And if you are not informed in detail, you have to communicate as close to the truth as possible.Physicians should be aware that more and more patients are demanding the truth, however cruel it may be. But when they refuse knowledge they may put the community, third parties, etc., at risk. E.g. AIDS, then the physician and the patient are obliged to receive and issue information as appropriate.

45- Are there limits to the duty to inform?

Information must be provided on the safe consequences, such as the loss of an organ and the risks that may occur with a certain degree of probability, according to scientific knowledge depending on the type of operation.

46- What should be excluded from the information?

Exceptional risks, i.e. risks that are not foreseeable to the best of scientific knowledge, may not be reported.

Information must be given if there is an express request from the patient. 48-Informed consent It is an authorisation given by the patient to undergo a specific medical procedure, i.e. an expression of his or her will.

It must always exist in writing.

Indispensable to be part of the medical record and given in advance.
necessary for better patient management and correct interpretation.

It should include: Diagnosis, chances of improvement or cure. Advantages and disadvantages of the practice to be carried out.

Possibilities of complications and possible alternative treatments.

Its non-existence by itself does not mean malpractice, but it is a background that will surely play against it in a lawsuit as it is highly valued by the judge.

49- Can the surgeon perform e.g. the removal of an organ that has not been removed?

Is such a possibility included in the informed consent? Regardless of what should be reported for a given intervention, it is also advisable to communicate about possible complications according to scientific information.

However, if there is an unexpected finding during the operation and the finding is life-threatening for the patient or seriously jeopardises her immediate future, the affected organ can be removed, detailing the findings and the reason for the removal in the surgical protocol which should be included in the medical record.

50- Is there anything more convincing to justify the surgeon?

Subsequently, the study of the excised part can support the determination.

The macroscopic view of the organ and the pathological anatomy may support the decision to remove what the surgeon considered indispensable, even if it was not included in the informed consent. For the judge, medical malpractice is an omissive conduct, contrary to the rules that impose a certain solicitous, attentive, shrewd behaviour. That is to say, who does not take the due precautions imposed by the circumstances of the case-Conf. Mosset Iturraspe according to Trigo Represas.

MYTHS ASSOCIATED WITH TRIALS OF MEDICAL LIABILITY

51- Are the trials due to bad medicine?

We do not believe that the trials are directly linked to bad medicine.

Today's medicine in general is far superior to times when trials of doctors were hardly exceptions.

In the US, the level of medicine in general is excellent and they have an excellent world record number of lawsuits against doctors and their health institutions.

52- Are the trials due to a few bad doctors?

This assessment is unfounded. Because obstetricians have many judgements against them, it does not mean that they are not professionally trained or are bad doctors.

We have seen distinguished professionals, heads of service, university professors, doctors of great prestige in the outside world, parade before the justice system.....

President Bush said: we must not forget a simple truth, that not every medical misfortune is the result of poor medicine, and nothing is risk-free. (The New York Times).

This is not to deny that malpractice cases exist.

53- Is only a university degree required to practice medicine?

No, with the diploma alone it is not possible.

Let's look at a practical example: the Province of Buenos Aires.

In this Province as in others with the title of doctor awarded by a medical State or private universities **are not allowed to practise medicine.**

In order to be able to do so, the bearer of the title is required by law to be compulsorily registered.

In a private body, in this case the Medical Associations, which, for a fee, actually allows the practice of medicine, e.g. in the Province of Buenos Aires.

Membership is not voluntary**, but compulsory**, as if the free election was a perished fact.

And we **reiterate** once again **that ethics has no owner**, but they shamelessly appropriate its banners.

54- Does insurance help to improve professional activity?

Health insurance does not enhance professional activity, it has a different function.

Doctors must be careful not to get caught up in the sense of security that they provide... I am sure of it. Perhaps this sensation experienced by some may lead to a decrease in attention in the development of their activity. Their existence in some cases may encourage lawsuits, since they those who make lawsuits know that there is financial backing and someone will pay.

There is no insurance in the world that can heal the wounds of a lawsuit, no matter how much you win.

55- Less than 50 years ago, lawsuits against the health care team were exceptional. Were they better doctors?

Patients in the first place have better information about their medical event through modern information systems and knowledge provided by technology that they did not have before.

They are also more aware of their rights and know that there is legislation in place to protect them.
protects.

Added to this is the increasingly complex feeling that man never wants to die and in most cases death happens as part of human nature independently of medical action.

On the other hand, old age is not accepted as a natural phenomenon of our lives.
species and claims eternal youth.

Plastic surgeons and the different techniques used to disguise the
The fact that they are old is proof of this.

It would seem that the health care team is responsible for death and for not providing eternal life.

These sensations have always existed, but exacerbated at this time and without the buffer of the old family doctor who accompanied his patient to death with his family.
This no longer exists, personalised medicine has been replaced by institutional medicine, where patients often do not even know the doctors and turn to the health centre they know best or the one closest to their home.

History also shows how variable societies and their inclinations are, you can fill a large Victorian square for a dictator and shortly afterwards fill it again in the name of democracy and freedom.

The examples in the world and in Argentina were very revealing in this respect, if honesty, freedom, freedom of speech, free thought, truth, free association are not valued. .... Why will doctors be respected?

56- Are lawsuits almost always won by patients?

This is not the case, trials are not won predominantly by the plaintiff.

57. After winning the case, the doctor returns to his or her normal routine.

Yes, but it leaves traces that are not easily forgotten, because even if you win the trial, you always lose, whether you lose a lot or a little, but you lose.

58- What do I lose if the trial is over and won?

A true myth as he may have been a victim during a long process of:

--Reactivation of pre-existing conditions

--Onset of new ailments as soon as you receive notification of the trial: anguish, depression, indifference, anger at what you consider an injustice, high blood pressure, diarrhoea, insomnia, bad mood, lack of appetite, decreased libido, dislike of the profession, resentment towards patients, thoughts of changing activities, shame in front of colleagues and own family. What do you explain to your teenage children, wife and friends?

Discredit, misunderstanding, indifference of their own colleagues, lack of
psychological support. Decreased income-Problems with insurance. Think about other activities within the specialty that are less risky.
So he finds his professional honour, self-esteem and self-confidence questioned.
prestige, the most important capital of professionals.

If you are close to retirement, retire or try administrative tasks.

These are some of the aspects observed, so you can win a lawsuit but often you cannot avoid the consequences, there are professionals who were not affected by the issue at all, although I think they are in the minority.

59- Is the psychophysical damage caused to doctors by the trials exaggerated?

J.Saxton and T.Leaman comment on the work of Sara C Charles MD psychiatrist at the University of Illinois-Chicago/American Journal of Psychiatry/

40% of the prosecuted doctors presented: depressive disorders including fatigue, gastrointestinal symptoms, insomnia, anorexia and headache, sense of defeat and frustration, as well as feeling useless and useless, bad mood.

The 20% in addition of the symptoms above felt difficulty from concentration, indecisiveness, feeling of anguish, irritability.

Eight per cent reported onset of new psychiatric conditions, including three physicians who suffered a myocardial infarction and 10 reported recrudescence of previous conditions.

Three doctors in the group studied were suicidal and four of them were
abused alcohol and drugs.

Only 6 had no demand-related symptoms.

Another group made changes in medical care, avoiding certain types of patients, making practices less compromising and other early retirement.

In other words, they actually took on negative aspects of defensive medicine while noting marital and child problems, Dr. Charles concluded in her study of defendant physicians.

60- Were all these trials avoidable?

More than 50% of prosecutions could have been avoided.

61- Are lawyers the real winners?

The only winners are the doctors who practised prevention, which is the system that gives the best results of all known systems.

62- I've already passed a trial, is my dose covered?

More than a few doctors have had more than one lawsuit. 63- Do lawyers encourage patients to litigate?
It is the patients and/or their relatives who knock on the lawyers' door

64- If several treatments are available and the doctor chooses one of them and the patient dies, is the judge interested in the outcome and does not care about the election?

The fact that there are several options and some discrepancy with the one used is not enough to hold the doctor guilty.

Guilt begins where scientific discussions end.

65- If I win the case, doesn't the patient have to pay anything?

To do so, you must have a benefit of litigation without costs with a favourable judgement.

66- Can't doctors have the benefit of no-expense-spared litigation?

If the necessary conditions of poverty are met, they can also get it. A house and a car are no impediment.

67- Can patients judge us and we cannot judge them?

If the judge rejected the claim as unfounded, malicious... the claim is sufficiently substantiated to be repeated against the plaintiff, i.e. the patient.

This practice should be better evaluated as it undoubtedly produced damage
to the professional.
68- Are there doctors who, because of their mistreatment and lack of concern during on-call duty of hospitals are assaulted?

The anguish caused by the illness, the pain, the long waiting times, the non-personalised treatment... produce in patients and relatives a degree of aggressiveness that is unjustly channelled towards the most vulnerable, which in this case is the doctor.

The latter has to pay for a health system that is still deficient, so that the intended recipient of the protest hardly ever appears.

However, violence, including insults, is never justifiable, as it is common for doctors in hospitals to be **the heroes of this pandemic. Lawyers are also insulted by the population.**

69-Without the benefit of no-cost litigation, no one litigates?

Approximately 85% have a no-cost litigation benefit, but there are other patients who have no objection to paying the court fee and other litigation costs, mainly in the crude cases where the outcome is estimated.

70- Do Codes of Ethics have practical application?

In Argentina, Codes of Ethics have moral value, but also legal relevance-O. Garay.

Doctrine of the Supreme Court of Justice of the Nation, ruling/Amante (JA- 1990-ll-125), which has given fundamental legal value to the moral norms that establish ethical duties for doctors, including this Code. For the doctor has a legal duty to act, not only on the basis of the obligation to act with prudence and full knowledge imposed by the rules of the Civil Code, but also as a consequence of the legal enforceability of the duty to assist the patient prescribed by the rules contained in the International Code of Medical Ethics and the Code of Ethics of the Argentine Medical Confederation and the Geneva Declaration.

71- Isn't a special medical mental health examination required for lawyers and doctors in any important role within their speciality?

Both lawyers and doctors can reach levels where people's freedom, property and honour depend on them, as well as doctors in health policies and heads of different specialties that directly affect the health of patients, as well as their own lives.

It is essential that all lawyers and doctors who aspire to higher office should have their mental condition examined as rigorously as possible.

This is done by companies for middle management, especially for people who
have so much responsibility for the lives of citizens.

It was not so long ago that we saw on TV a legislator with a quasi-sexual scene in Argentina, which forced the Speaker of the House to suspend the session while a law was being discussed.

Would this legislator have withstood a regular psychic examination?

There is no doubt, given the obvious facts, that not only doctors and lawyers should have their psychological sphere examined when they aspire to higher positions, but also to high positions such as legislators, President of the Nation, Ministers, etc. etc. It is essential that they **guarantee their psychological integrity** to citizens.

In order not to give local examples that could be misinterpreted, we ask ourselves, can anyone think that Hitler, Mussolini, Stalin, Mao, Putin, the African dictators .... and Americans... would have passed a psychic examination? It is simply an indispensable act of prevention.

Logically, a psychological test that is not normal **disqualifies one from applying for any position of medium responsibility, and it is those who sign the aptitude test who are responsible, as well as those who ignore the recommendations of unsuitability and approve the appointments.**

72- Are judges and doctors addicted?

I don't know the statistics, but we assume that they have the same levels as the general population, but they are hidden, protected by their co-workers and when they come to light then it is too late. It is a false protection. There are medical specialties that are more exposed.

Argentina is the third country in the Americas in alcohol consumption, mainly among young people.

73- The surgeon responsible for postoperative follow-up should be the surgeon who operated?

The surgeon is responsible for the surgical procedure, but the general responsibility lies with the anaesthesiologist, who are historically the founders of modern intensive care and who know the problems of the postoperative period and its imbalances.

This is reasonable for common interventions, where there are highly complex operations, patients go directly to the intensive care unit.

The world's first Intensive Care Unit as it is known today was established in 1953 by Bjorn Ibsep, a Danish anaesthesiologist, who is considered the father of intensive care and his Intensive Care Unit was located at the Copenhagen Community Hospital.

The first scientific paper on Intensive Care was published in the journal Nordisk Medicin, Norway in 1958 under the title: The work in an anesthesiologist Observation Unit, authored by Bjorn together with the Danish anesthesiologist Tone Dahil Kvittingen. Baltimore anaesthesiologist, teacher and researcher Peter Safar, who was active as early as 1958, was considered the father of modern cardiopulmonary resuscitation.

In 1972, the Australian Society of Anaesthesiologists initiated the publication of Anahesthesia and Intensive Care.

74- Are ethics compatible with the economic interests of a medical institution where business is the priority?

Ethics is the best long-term success insurance for any company, as it makes its products credible and trustworthy.

75- Can any doctor have a trial?

Undoubtedly, but it is not difficult to observe how, on occasion, judgements are made in favour of a certain group of professionals clearly identified by the establishment's management as possible candidates. Although there are patients whose objective in litigation is profit, no one can deny that medical, dental, etc. malpractice exists, although in cases of serious medical malpractice only a small number of patients resort to justice, and if they make up 15% of the injured parties, that is a lot to say.

And there are no more lawsuits because there are trial lawyers who don't litigate for
litigate and guard their prestige by not sponsoring legal adventures.

76- Can there be a contract between doctor and patient if there is nothing signed? In May 1936 the French Court of Cassation already stated that a contract is formed between a doctor and a patient if there is nothing signed.
between doctor and patient a real contract and that the involuntary violation of the
The latter was sanctioned by a liability of the same nature.

There is a real contract with obligations of the parties as explained above without any signature and it is formalised with the start of the medical care.

77- Does all cosmetic surgery represent an obligation of result?

Topic already developed in another point to which we can add a ruling of the National

Chamber of Appeals in Civil Matters - Chamber 5 of 8/4/2008 which among other things says:

There is a rule, usually not unknown to the patient, according to which the expected result may not be achieved even though the doctor has taken the greatest possible care in the operation. Law 17.132 art. 20 inc. 1 and 2 does not make any distinction according to the type of operation, so that in all cases **an obligation of means is assumed, without ruling out the existence of risks.**

The medical team

78- Is the surgical team leader responsible for everything that happens in the operating theatre?

The surgeon, in this case, was historically the captain of the ship, but the law gradually turned to almost put the institution as the responsible head.

Medicine is ceasing to be an individual act and becoming a collective activity, as in the case of a surgical intervention, the judge will encounter a problem **of anonymity** and difficulty in locating the member of the team that has caused harm.

At the same time, some of the members of the surgical team have **scientific autonomy**, so that the chief surgeon at that moment has no responsibility, as he does not know about anaesthesia, extracorporeal circulation etc. and these members of the team will have their own personal responsibility.

The surgeon has responsibility for what he or she can control or supervise.

For example, if the anaesthesiologist leaves the operating theatre to talk on the phone, he/she will undoubtedly share responsibility, as he/she was able to control and supervise that event.

It should be borne in mind that individual liability never disappears and there can be plural liability.

79- Is there no solution to identify any member given the number of doctors in the team?

This problem can be solved in many cases with an adequate delimitation of roles, differentiation and coordination of the competences and obligations of each of the members.

This will further limit the responsibility of the chief surgeon in the case of classic surgical intervention.

80- Does the division of labour contribute?It can be of great help in clarifying this issue.

81- When does the division of labour fail?

When the selection of collaborators is not correct. When communication between team members fails With imperfect coordination.
General organisational failures

82- Is it in the interest of the prosecuted doctor that the lawsuit be criminal?

Liability is the consequence of an event in which an individual is injured.
interest protected by law.

When the consequence of such non-compliance results in a penalty, it is criminal liability.

If compensation is required, the liability is civil liability, which may be contractual or non-contractual.

Criminal liability **is personal and non-transferable**, the guilty party must serve the sentence and also everything is extinguished by death.

In civil liability, one is liable with one's assets, with all present and future assets.

On his death the property passes to his heirs passing on the responsibility.

Furthermore, we can say that in criminal law **it is not the institutions that are imprisoned** but the persons, and in civil law the compensation is always patrimonial.

In criminal law, however, the evidence that the judge needs to convict must be strong and concrete, a reasonable requirement since nothing less than a person's liberty is at stake.

That is why it is always more viable for the plaintiff to take the civil rather than the criminal route, although this route can be useful even if he knows that he will not win in order to have some quick proof without much effort.

In any case, **there are** logically **more judgements unfavourable to doctors in the civil sphere than in the criminal sphere.**

83- Should Codes of Ethics be made by medical institutions? Lorenzetti, Luis Ricardo, member of the Supreme Court of Justice of the United States of America.
Argentine Nation, argues that: However, it is interesting to note that a possible medicalisation of the legal system, since if it confers on the colleges the power to dictate codes of ethics and regulatory norms that are valid for third parties, the regulation of the activity is left in their hands. In our opinion, ethics has no specific owner.

84- Is there any impediment for the secretary to complete the list of medicines on a prescription previously signed by me, if she already knows the patient?

This is a bad habit and can lead to severe problems that the
The doctor will not be able to disengage as it is signed by him.

This applies to other functions that are entrusted to the secretary or non-medical assistant. On the other hand, leaving signed prescriptions is an important imprudence that can have any unpleasant consequence.

85- Is it reasonable for the patient to send me a refrigerator and a dishwasher from his business instead of paying money for the operation?

Bartering is a thing of the past, but it is in good taste to avoid such situations, as it would seem to be an act of trade.

86Should the medical fees be adjusted according to the severity of the ailment?

The CNCiv .Sala E Argentina, opportunely said that they will depend on the intensity of the treatment, seriousness of the illness, fortune of the patient... The CNCiv, Chamber F Argentina It ruled that the fees also depend on the success of the operation, the patient's financial situation and the post-operative care provided by the surgeon.

The CNCiv D said: the fees also depend on the characteristic of the ailment. Chamber B adds to the statements that the fees also depend on success. obtained

On a personal note, nothing could be more **unseemly, discriminatory and totally far removed from being a doctor and which would disgust Marañón himself by** linking medical fees according to the patient's fortune, the success of the operation, whether the surgeon attended to the postoperative period, the seriousness of the ailment, the intensity of the treatment, prestige.... If, before landing at Barajas, the pilot has to negotiate a major storm front, turn away and then land in strong side winds and succeed in landing, the flight attendant would indicate to the passengers on deplaning that they must pay extra fees for the severity of the storm, the economic position of each passenger and for the success of the landing in the face of situations such as those experienced during the storm.

If in a taxi the driver charges you extra when there is a lot of traffic, when you arrive successfully at your destination and also because you took it at the corner of a bank, you assume that you are a man of wealth....

What would you, judges and doctors of prestige think?

87- Do I get paid first, then trade?

It's like buying a fridge, first the supermarket charges for it and then I take it away.

There are particular situations where the operation requires materials to be purchased in advance, in these cases it is reasonable to request money in advance.

The example is extreme, but they are similar in some ways. The doctor in his defence must consider /see ut supra/ that there are no longer patients but consumers, and if the doctor charges in advance, everything can be transformed into an act of commerce.

As we can see in this specific case, we are walking along a cobbled road with large potholes. This is an issue that should be debated and studied in detail.

CONSCIENTIOUS OBJECTION

88- What is Conscientious Objection?

It is a form of non-compliance with the law, whose essential characteristic is that the rule is rejected only insofar as it affects the subject personally, as a form of protection of his individual freedom, so that the objector does not seek with his objection to modify or do away with the rule (M. Blazquez-J. Calvin).

In other words, when compliance with the norm is at odds with issues of
religious, moral, ethical, etc. 89- What is the legal basis?
The reference is to Articles 14 and 19 of the National Constitution, which guarantee freedom of worship, freedom of conscience and freedom of action not to harm third parties.

Human rights covenants with constitutional status

Universal Declaration of Human Rights, freedom of conscience is protected by Article 18 of the Universal Declaration of Human Rights.

San José, Costa Rica, Article 12 (freedom of conscience and religion).

Article 6 of Law 26130.Conscientious Objection. Any person, whether a physician or auxiliary personnel of the health system, has the right to exercise conscientious objection without any labour consequences....

Article 10 of Law 27610 states: The health professional who must directly intervene in the termination of a pregnancy has the right to exercise conscientious objection. ....

Italian Constitutional Court/1991:...it is an inalienable right of everyone.
men...

90- When does Conscientious Objection not apply?

In emergency cases where the life of the person is in danger, the physician must act, even if he or she must act on an abortion that has already been performed.

91- Essential conditions?

The objector must inform in advance what his or her conduct will be.

The objector must have the same conduct in private or state activity.

92- Should advance notice be given?

Indispensable, there is no special format but the writing must be clear and legible. E.g.:

Reports on Conscientious Objection

Date

Mr. Director of ....

José Antonio ...., in my capacity as a doctor of the Institution .... I hereby declare my Conscientious Objection, refusing to carry out any abortive procedure or similar processes because they affect my most intimate and deepest personal ethical and religious convictions, while exercising my right to freedom of conscience, without affecting the rights of the patient.

You are hereby formally notified of my decision Signature/complaint/address/telephone/email. This should be done in duplicate and the copy signed by the
and with the date of submission.

93- Misuse of conscientious objection

Conscientious objection is an individual, personal act which, although it has antecedents, has been updated in Argentina since Law 27610, which authorises the interruption of pregnancy.

Physicians and auxiliary personnel have every right to take refuge under this protective mantle whenever the law violates their strongest conscientious and religious convictions.

It may happen that the physician misuses it as a deferral, an impediment or an excuse to proselytise his or her ideas, and it may be an obstacle that keeps him or her from the real right that legitimately belongs to him or her.

In addition to any of these attitudes being ethically incorrect, an action for protection can be brought against the healthcare establishment and the doctor himself (Article 43 CN) and also gives rise to legal liability as it may involve wilful breach of professional duties (art.1724 CCyC)..... wilful misconduct is caused by intentionally causing damage or with manifest disregard for the interests of others.

94- How is a referral made for a patient whose doctor did not perform an abortion on the grounds of conscientious objection?

A situation that can be conflictive when the objector refuses to refer her to another doctor or institution, since the objector would be acting against his own conscience by cooperating with an action that he considers immoral, so that he is not obliged to facilitate the abortion, since his conduct is protected by the same right that allows him to defend his status as an objector, although his situation is complicated.

On the other hand, how does the doctor know where the right place is?
to refer the patient?

Do you have to have a register of clinics and/or doctors and know their qualifications?

Does it become a necessary party to the abortion?

Can referring her to a particular institution cause him to be liable for malpractice and death at the point of referral?

95- What should be the referral mechanism?

The competent authority should leave a list of clinics or doctors for referral as far in advance as possible at the establishment where the doctor is treating the patient. Such specific and time-consuming matters cannot be delegated to one clinic alone.

Another less desirable solution is for the institution where the doctor works to have and communicate the places that can receive the patient and the administrative employee will refer her on the indication of the objecting doctor.

96- Can institutions exercise the right to conscientious objection?
e.g. not to carry out abortions?

Sanatoriums do not have an institutional conscience like human beings, so this possibility can be denied. This is the central argument of those who oppose this right of institutions.

However, there are hospitals and sanatoriums that belong to religious orders or that publicly profess a particular faith, and as such are in a position to apply for conscientious objection for their institution. Council of Europe Resolution 1763:...**no person, hospital or institution shall be coerced, held civilly liable or discriminated against on account of its refusal to authorise, participate in or assist in the performance of an abortion for any reason whatsoever.**

97- Are there countries where the conscientious objection of health care institutions is respected? Uruguay, France ,42 US States ...

98- Side effect for objecting doctors.

The objecting physician must be vigilant as in some cases it is possible that measures may be taken that may be detrimental to his or her professional development or work.

99- Does conscientious objection under Article 10 of the law extend to the professionals necessary for the performance of an abortion, anaesthesiologists, nurses, instrumentalists and other personnel involved in the operation?

Article 10 /see ut supra/ has the professional as the main actor and nothing is said about the necessary auxiliary personnel, or at least it is not explicit, so that it is not taken into account by the law.

On a personal level it would seem to be a discriminatory measure, as auxiliary staff should also be protected by law as they are part of the same process.

See Article 6 of Law 26130 and other international treaties. It is accepted from the point of view of the law that auxiliaries have the same right as the acting physician to request conscientious objection / nurses, instrumentalist-anaesthesiologist.../

Ethics and religious principles, along with personal convictions, are
the objector's livelihood.

The entire team involved in an abortion operation has a legitimate interest in the
right to have their will respected and to be able to be an objector.

Residents may fall into the category of objectors if they are sent to
perform an abortion.

On a different note, it seems prudent to differentiate between what is a
civil disobedience and conscientious objection.

The former is a political and collective action, while conscientious objection is individual, ethical and conscientious.

What is the legal effect? Exonerating the physician and the intervening team from performing an act that they would otherwise be obliged to perform, abortion being the classic example.

Of course, faced with a doctor's conscientious objection, a woman may, in the case of abortion, object to medical care that is in principle guaranteed to her by the established legal order.

PSYCHIATRIC HOSPITALISATION INVOLUNTARY

100- What should a doctor know when intervening in an involuntary psychiatric hospitalisation?

Enforcing the law

Article 28

Mental health admissions should be in general hospitals,
This is what Article 28 of the law says.

To this end, public network hospitals must be provided with the resources necessary.

101- If the internment is refused?

The refusal of outpatient or inpatient care for the sole reason of mental health problems shall be considered a discriminatory act under the terms of law 23592.

102- Does the hospitalisation have to be notified?

The competent judge and the Review Body must be notified within 10 hours of the duly founded involuntary internment, and all the evidence provided for in Article 20 must be added within 48 hours at the latest.

103- What are the obligations of the judge in Argentina?

The judge, within a maximum of 3 calendar days of being notified, must:

a- Authorise, if it assesses that the grounds provided for by this law are met

b- To request additional reports from the treating professionals or to indicate external expert opinions, provided that they do not harm the evolution of the treatment, in order to assess whether the necessary assumptions exist to justify the extreme measure of involuntary internment.

c- Deny in case it is assessed that the necessary assumptions for the measure of internment do not exist, in which case it must ensure immediate discharge.

104- What are the injunctions?

Article 24 of the Mental Health Act

Having authorised involuntary commitment, the judge must request reports at intervals of no more than 30 calendar days in order to reassess whether the reasons for the continuation of such a measure persist and may at any time order immediate removal.

If after the first 90 days and after the third report the involuntary placement continues, the judge shall ask the Review Body to appoint an interdisciplinary team that has not been involved so far and if possible independent of the intervening health care service in order to obtain a new assessment,

In the event of a difference of criteria, it shall always opt for the least restrictive one. the freedom of the detained person

105-Legal action after 7 days of hospitalisation.

Article 25 of the law provides that after the first 7 days in the case of involuntary interventions, the judge shall report to the Review Body.

106- What is the Review Body?

This is provided for in Article 38 of the law when it states that the Review Body is created within the Public Defender's Office with the aim ofprotecting the human rights of users of mental health services.

107- What are the specific functions of this Review Body?

1- Collect information to assess the conditions under which treatment is being carried out
2- For this reason it must be multidisciplinary
3- Monitor in-patient conditions
4- Assess that involuntary hospitalisations are duly justified and that they do not last longer than necessary.
5- Control that the derivations are in the correct conditions.
set out in Article 30 of the law.
6- Inform the enforcement authority
7- Requesting judicial intervention in irregular situations
8- Make proposals and modifications.

108. Can visits to a boarding school be prevented?

In principle, no. But there are exceptions

109- If there is a limitation, must the judge be aware of it? The judge must be informed and know the reasons.

110- Does this limitation apply to the defence counsel?

The limitation does not apply to the defence counsel. 111 Does the prisoner have the right to a defence counsel? Yes, if he does not appoint one, the State must provide one.

112- Abandonment of the place of internment

In voluntary internment, the interned person may leave the institution. It is limited only if there is a risk to the patient himself or to third parties. 113- Hospitalisation against the patient's will
It is not possible within our regulations.

In cases of gravity and/or urgency, actions for injunctive relief can be brought and the judge shall decide.

If in an insanity proceeding, the judge decides to disqualify himself. The solution is the same as that of a doctor who decides not to treat such a patient any more. He must continue until another colleague or institution replaces him so as not to leave him without medical care.

The same applies to the judge, as he cannot leave the child in a helpless situation, but must continue until the child is handed over to another judge.

114- In which cases can he/she be committed against his/her will?

Only when the health care team determines that there is a situation of
certain or close risk for the patient and for third parties. And that there is no other possibility of effective treatment.
Recalling that detention must be notified within 10 hours to the judge and the Review Body.

RESPONSIBILITY OF DENTISTS AND NURSES

115- It is the doctor, not the nurse, who is responsible for the patient.

The nurse's responsibility is governed by the same rules as that of physicians and has specific responsibilities as his or her actions are autonomous.

116- What can he be accused of?

He or she may act with impudence, recklessness or negligence, and can also be
The Commission is not responsible for the non-compliance with the rules governing its activity.

117- Can the care facility be blamed for some of the above-mentioned non-compliance?

Their guilt will drag down the health institution and in some cases the doctor who should have taken supervisory action.

118- What are the possibilities for nurse error or mistake?
1- Error in the drug as well as in the dosage.
2- Error in patient identification, giving the medication to another person
person who does not belong.
3- Failure to properly supervise falls, bedsores...
4- Errors in the use of appliances
5- Poor compliance with medical orders
6- Poor quality communication with the doctor
7- Failure to properly record what was done.
8- Medication on your own
9- Failure to report observed irregularities

The role of the nurse is extremely important and irreplaceable. He is more in contact with the hospitalised patient and his relatives than the doctor himself. And he/she has to respond at times which goes beyond his/her possibilities when there are doubts left for the patient and/or relatives.

Deserves special training to manage patient and family relations as well as possible. Many family members know the name of the nurse and do not remember the name of the doctor.
119- Do dentists have the same level of responsibility as dentists in the doctors?

They are governed by the same legal and ethical standards as physicians.

Their judgements are clearly on the increase. 120-Type of obligation of dentists Dentists have an obligation of means just like doctors. Obligations of result are rare. Rulings: The provision of dental care is an obligation of means and not of result, as it does not guarantee the recovery of the assisted person, but rather the appropriate treatment, with a commitment to prudent care.

Another ruling from the year 2000 The failure to achieve an expected result in a dental treatment does not necessarily lead to the attribution of liability to the practitioner, since success is conditioned by the interaction of various circumstances...

In the same year: The obligation assumed by the dentist with regard to implants is one of result, as the patient undergoes such treatment in search of a result typical of aesthetic surgeries.

We respectfully disagree with this latest ruling, provided that the practitioner has taken all the steps required by dental science in such cases.

121-What should be recommended to a dentist?

1- Do not go beyond your technical, instrumental and assistants' possibilities.
in the practices in his office.

2- Do not perform anaesthesia or sedation in your own practice if you are not qualified to do so, and certainly not on your own.

3- If the surgery is authorised for surgical practices use
always to an anaesthesiologist.

4- The clinical history should follow the same guidelines as the one taken
by doctors, which is not always the case.

5- You should be aware of the diseases that patients are suffering from and what is their medication.

6- In case you have to evacuate a patient the ambulance stretcher may not fit in the lift, have it as an issue of concern.

7- Have a basic understanding of resuscitation.

8- Have keep in mind hat the anaesthesia local anaesthesia can have atsometimes have general repercussions.

As there is a contract between the dentist and his injured patient for the provision of services by the former to the latter, the liability that may be incurred on that basis can only be contractual, arising from the breach of the obligations thus assumed. It is contractual liability for the fact of things, based on an implicit duty of security or guarantee on the part of the person who has delivered a thing or makes use of it for the fulfilment of its performance, if the same later results in damage that is linked to obligations arising from the contract (from the dissenting vote of Dr. Azpelicueta).Capel.CC Junín 20/4/1988.Seta de Etchevers, Rosa c/Gesuiti Jorge y otro, Rep LL 1988-528, sum 132. Although subsequent changes in legislation have nothing to do with it, the dental and medical relationship has been considered to be contractual in nature since those years. Nurses who are required to provide important services to doctors, given the training they receive to obtain their diploma, are empowered to appreciate elementary circumstances of patient care on their own initiative.... Mendoza de Lallera, Adelfina J v. Municipality of Buenos Aires et al.

MEDICINE DEFENSIVE

122-What is defensive medicine?

The harassed physician, fearful of being sued, takes defensive measures at his or her discretion.

Some practitioners argue strongly that not preparing to fight is preparing to fall.

For this he has a weapon and he believes it to be highly effective: the pen, his pencil.

In order for the judge to see, in the event of being sued, that the obligations of means are sufficiently fulfilled.

Excessive requests for laboratory tests, various crude and non-crucial practices such as imaging tests...and how much more can be asked of a patient.

The aim is to make the judge think, everything that has been done to care for the patient in the best possible way, there is almost nothing left to do, as even the discharge takes a little longer than necessary, just in case.

He sometimes forgets that the first medical act is to shake the patient's hand when he enters the office, and if possible, to call him by name before taking the pen.

The handshake 5,000 years ago was used by the Egyptians to seal acts and arrangements between men as a way of guaranteeing compliance.

Practising defensive medicine is a double mistake, since it is not synonymous with better medicine and secondly because the judge knows how to distinguish.

We know that it is not always easy to differentiate between the necessary and the superfluous, as sometimes there is a fine line between the two.

So it is not easy to calculate the costs of defensive medicine, which is why not many authors have been able to pinpoint the method of calculating them.

Surely our estimates, we consider that they do not have a mathematical accuracy, but conceptual and quite close to reality. 123Does this practice harm the patient?

It can only harm you when you are repeatedly exposed to lightning or have to bear the risks of an instrumental examination, loss of time, etc.

124- Who is harmed by this behaviour?

This is a job we ask the reader to do their own calculations to answer at what level injury occurs. This presentation has **this practical work** as part of the training exercise, which is indispensable at this point.

125- Cost of defensive medicine

Start of the practical exercise.

It is of singular importance that doctors, lawyers, judicial, public health and political authorities expand and improve this exercise, or devise a practical formula to calculate it with more precision and scientific rigour.

A possible calculation plan with approximate figures.

Number of doctors in Argentina: **Let's assume there are 200,000** doctors to make round numbers.

10% do not see patients, as they are engaged in other medical activities, so they do not practise care medicine.

Therefore: 200,000 - 20,000 = **180,000 doctors.**

Of this number who see patients, 70% of them practice defensive medicine in some form.

That leaves **126,000**.

To continue, it is necessary to know how many patients each doctor sees per day.

Not all of these patients leave with a prescription or medical order that will affect defensive medicine, only 3 of the possible 8 e.g. you will see on the day.

This leaves **3 patients** who leave with a prescription ordering
the different practices motivated by defensive medicine.

Multiply the number o f doctors left practising defensive medicine by 3 and you have the number of prescriptions per day for the entire mass of doctors.

Therefore the 126.000 doctors x 3 patients per day=378.000
This is the number of patients per day who receive some kind of indication for pharmacological, laboratory, imaging or instrumental examinations, cardiology, etc. from general practitioners and specialists involved in defensive medicine.

Multiply this daily number by 275 which is the annual number of days worked and you will have the annual number, being the final number of patients seen who leave with a prescription affected by Defensive Medicine....

It remains to assess what is the superfluous cost of the over-prescribed to multiply it by the above result obtained, which in each country will be different.

Think then of the cost of all the imaging tests, laboratory possibilities, cardiological studies with all their variants, interconsultations, endoscopies, prolongation of hospitalisation days, etc. etc. etc. etc. etc.It remains to put the approximate figure of over-performance for each patient, each
one will take into account the market price of the various practices. It is estimated at $12 of over-benefit for each patient in Argentina, which varies from month to month. This final result is multiplied by that $12 and gives a figure that is divided by the GDP for the year and multiplied by 100 to get the final number for the cost of defensive medicine.

This will show what percentage of GDP corresponds to spending caused by defensive medicine.In Argentina, spending decreased significantly and it is estimated that approximately 0.20% of GDP for the year.

So **0.20** is the approximate percentage of GDP wasted on Defensive Medicine in Argentina despite the positive change in this area.

Overall expenditure was taken, without differentiatingmedicine private,state, institutional etc.

This is a really high figure, but it does not mean that this expenditure will lead to better quality medicine.

On the other hand, it is an invitation to those interested in the subject to ratify, modify, rectify, disqualify, expand..... these numbers y concepts as they do not have the necessary scientific rigour to consider these figures as benchmarks, but they are not so far removed from reality.

In other respects, the costs of defence medicine in Argentina are not very different from those incurred in developed countries.

The figures taken as a reference can be widely variable as in May 2023 the MONTHLY inflation in Argentina was 7.8 % and the INTERANNUAL inflation was over 114.2 %.

These figures mean that those taken for this exercise can lend themselves to confusion and be highly variable.

The percentages of physicians practising defensive medicine in Argentina were taken from a survey conducted in the provinces of Entre Ríos, Corrientes, Buenos Aires, Mendoza, Santa Fe and the city of Buenos Aires, following presentations on medical liability.

It is a survey which, although it coincides with European and US countries, does not have the necessary scientific rigour, as it is very complicated to put exact figures, especially with the variants that Argentina presents.

There is a clear link between this significant expenditure and medical liability lawsuits.

This calculation did not take into account the increased number of staff required to meet this over-provision, nor the cost of reagents and equipment, nor the time spent by doctors and other members of the health team in different practices, the waiting period for patients....

Also not counted were professionals who retire before the corresponding time and changes in their speciality for lower-risk tasks.

Costs in the US

The cost of medical issues related to the trials and all that surrounds them.
was so important that it forced Congress to look deeper into the issue.
It accounted for 20% of the final cost of all health care in that country. It also accounted for 20% of total health care spending in the State of Texas.
health care in 1994.

126- Some significant items

The unconscionable lab and cabinet indication alone accounted for 8% of the US health budget, equivalent to $10 billion.

In the same country, the amount requested for mild head injuries in people aged 5-24 years in imaging examinations together with cervical spine was considered exaggerated, as the expenditure amounted to 45 million dollars per year (Horacio Canto).

We refer to the publication of Vasanthakumar N. Bath.Ed. Auburn House of his book Medical Malpractice/ Comprehensive Analysis which can give us a clear idea of the magnitude of the problem at hand.

127- What are the historical costs?

As always, the USA is the country of comparison and the leader in the field.
of malpractice suits worldwide (by the same author).

The total cost of malpractice for all items was 13.7 billion
dollars in 1984 in that country.

Defensive medicine accounted for 4.3 trillion of this total cost.

This date is taken because in that five-year period the growth in the number of lawsuits in The US suffered a large increase.

Although projected to 1998 it was estimated at 15.17 billion. 128- Is there a link between caesarean sections and defensive medicine?
The Pan American Health Organization informs us that 4 out of every 10 deliveries result in caesarean births.

The same organisation reports that the ideal is one caesarean section every ten years. births.

129- In Argentina, is there a difference between the state and the private sector in the practice of caesarean section?

In the field of public health, it is estimated that between 25% and 35% of the births are by caesarean section,In the private sector the percentage ranges between 50% and 75%. In Argentina, the number provided by the WHO is three times higher.
130- What is the number of caesarean sections considered ideal by the WHO?

In 2015, the WHO considered the ideal caesarean section rate to be between
10 and 15 % of all births. In Argentina we triple the figures.
131- Is the increase in the number of unscheduled caesarean sections directly related to the linked to defensive medicine?

This question led us to consult obstetricians, lawyers specialising in the subject and directors of clinics in the greater Buenos Aires area, and some conclusions were reached, many of which coincide with the non-medical view of the subject.

a- Between 13-15% of women prefer caesarean section to natural childbirth and put pressure on the obstetrician in the name of patient autonomy and directly request it.

b- The aim is to avoid the pain of childbirth.

c- Previous caesarean section and pre-existing conditions.

d- A few of them lose only a couple of hours, when in a normal delivery they can spend more than 12 hours in the sanatorium, an important issue if they work in several centres.

e- Obstetricians are reaching the podium of medical liability lawsuits, which is why at the slightest difficulty, they decide not to risk anything, and indicate the operation.

This is a typical measure of defensive medicine.

There is a serious risk of generalisation on this issue, as Argentina has a medical corps with the same level of professionalism as in first world countries, albeit with insufficient technology.Defensive medicine is not an Argentine invention.

There is no doubt that lawsuits against the medical profession do not only harm those directly concerned, but are projected onto society as a whole, including, of course, the patients.

Not much effort is seen to point doctors in other directions than this misguided way of defending themselves.

The range of figures is likely to be variable, but there is no doubt thatat least for developing countries such as Argentina, it is a number huge and ruthless that is not properly explored in depth for its study and solution.

THE MEDICAL ERROR

132- Is the error not punishable?

Iturraspe and Lorenzetti in Medical Contracts explain the trend that appreciates that modern life is not error-free. Tunc goes on to say that a good family man cannot speak without offending grammar, cannot play tennis without missing balls and, according to statistics, this good family man makes nine mistakes for every five minutes of urban traffic. The error is punishable when one acts without knowing the patient well or when one carries out practices that are at odds with the lex artis.

133- Is it punishable for minor offences?

We consider that error may not be punishable in minor offences.

Not every mistake is to blame

134- What do judges say about medical error?

Garay O in his Code cites:

The simple error of diagnosis or treatment is not enough to give rise to compensable damage, because in a branch of knowledge in which opinion is the predominant matter of opinion, it is difficult to set precise limits between what is right and what is wrong.

CNCiv, Chamber B, 22/12/1964,LL118-923/12.207,/SJ-Buenos Aires

The diagnostic error is not imputable if all measures have been taken to avoid it and no ignorance of the subject matter has been revealed, and no more can be demanded of the doctor than can be demanded of the average doctor, unless he is a specialist.

CNCiv, Chamber A, 29/07/1977, ED, 74-563-Buenos Aires

The diagnostic error, in order to be considered as a factor attributable to the doctor, must be due to a gross assessment, negligence or lack of skill in the investigation of the causes of the illness, ruling out this circumstance, the simple error of diagnosis or treatment, which is not sufficient to generate the obligation to pay compensation, because in a branch of knowledge where opinion is predominant, it is difficult to establish the contours to limit what is correct and what is not. It is therefore necessary to the usual degree of skill and diligence common to members of his or her profession. C1CC

Are there statistics in Argentina?

I am not aware of their existence, but we know, for example, that in the USA, the Washington Academy of Sciences in its study entitled /Errar is Human/ explains that they are the fifth leading cause of death in that country.

From the same work they report that about 100,000 people die annually as a result of errors, imperfection, recklessness and negligence and that it means an expenditure of 29 billion dollars. We interpret this figure as corresponding to all cases linked to medical failure.

How do doctors view the justice system? They find it contradictory, frustrating and intimidating, with the latter agreeing with the latter.
vision with doctors from other countries.

137- Is it the medical expert who reports whether there was negligence?

The existence of negligence in the medical action is ruled by the judges
and the medical expertise can be taken as a reference. 138- When is the error punishable?
It is punishable when the necessary measures were not taken to clarify diagnoses, when inter-consultations were not carried out, when the necessary means were not exhausted in the face of doubt or simple suspicion. If a general practitioner refers a patient to a specialist, he/she has the obligation to think that he/she was sent for a reason and to pay the utmost attention.

Of course, the error of a specialist has a higher connotation of seriousness. Of course, inexperience is punishable, as is negligence.

The Joint Commission on Accreditation of Health Care Organisation promotes a culture of error recognition as the surest way to reduce errors.

It is practised by 30 states in the USA**: Im sorry laws**, without being synonymous with guilt.

Bello Janeiro says that when the appropriate measures for diagnosis and treatment are applied and the appropriate tests are carried out, the orientation of the diagnosis to an inaccurate judgement does not imply liability on its own.

Nor is the practitioner making a diagnostic error when the patient does not shows definite signs of pathology.

The law is interested in knowing the causes of the error, in order to be able to judge. There are also errors that occur when the patient does not report correctly or only partially or not at all, or does not report anything that could be of unique diagnostic value. In these cases the professional can explain the causes of the error.The Spanish Ministry of Health and Consumer Affairs reported that medication errors affected 4% of all hospitalised patients.

This is a broader chapter linked to errors

In the US, medication errors result in at least one death daily and approximately 1.3 million people are harmed annually. Every minute 5 patients die from medical errors. United Nations.
15% of hospital expenditure in the countries of the Organisation were
related to the topic.

This is the third time that WHO is organising a global Patient Safety Challenge declaring 17 September 2022 as Patient Safety Day. World Health Assembly, resolution WHA 72.6

In 1999, To Err is Human was published by the Committee on Quality of Health Care in America-Institute of Medicine with figures related to medical error that are surprising in their magnitude. Error is the third leading cause of death in the USA, British Medical Journal 2016.

ASSISTED REPRODUCTION

139- What control do establishments working in reproduction have? assisted?

Resolution 1305/15 of the National Ministry of Health approved the rules for the authorisation and control of gamete banks, i.e. spermatozoa and oocytes, and establishes the obligation to store them in two separate places.

The bank should have duplicate records of its donors, sample destinations and recipients.

140Is the father the sperm donor?

Article 558 of the new Civil Code is clear: they are children of the person who gave birth and of the man or woman who gave consent, as long as this consent is duly registered in the Civil Registry, regardless of who provided the gametes or embryos,

141-Requirements for birth registration

It must be stated in the corresponding basic file for birth registration that the person was born by assisted reproduction technique with gametes from a third party, and that at the request of the latter, information on the donor's medical data may be obtained from the intervening Health Centre when it is relevant to the health of the donor.

142Donor anonymity is total?

The identity of the donor may be disclosed for duly substantiated reasons assessed by a judicial authority.

143- Do children have the right to know their genetic background? They have the right to know their genetic origin.
144- Can parentage be contested?

It is not possible to challenge the parentage of a person who has provided the corresponding consent.

In any case, the donor did not give his willingness to exercise filiation.

We must bear in mind that it is unacceptable to recognise, exercise
of any action or claim of filial relationship in respect of the gamete donor.

145- Is the donor sperm screened?
Measures should be taken to ensure that congenital diseases or pathologies are not transmitted. Remembering that in principle the identity of the donor must be safeguarded.

The physician shall not inseminate if preservation is unlikely.
of secrecy or suspicion of illness.

146- Does the donor have a monetary acknowledgement? It must be free of charge
147- What is the husband's right?

Where the insemination has been carried out with the consent of the husband, the child shall be considered as the legitimate child of the wife and husband and no one may dispute paternity on the sole ground that insemination has been carried out.

148- Is it possible to claim maintenance from the sperm donor?

No action for maintenance may be brought against the donor.

149- Is there any risk of transmitting diseases or congenital malformations?

The risk exists, albeit limited. 150-Unmarried mother
If your partner has given consent you cannot escape your responsibility for the child, unless you can prove that the child was not born by artificial insemination.

151- Medical collection

The physician performing this procedure must be confident that the medical, legal and social implications of the procedure are fully understood, and receive written authorisation.

PATIENT RIGHTS

152- Has there been legislation in this direction for greater patient protection? in the face of medical activity?

The legislation is in line with the already established concepts of patients' rights linked to the respect of their will and life decisions. In any case, it ratified the rights installed to date.

153- Was the patient medically unprotected prior to the law providing for his or her rights?

In no way can it be interpreted that legislation has been passed to protect patients from alleged medical abuses, which in fact never existed, but rather to update and legalise certain behaviours that are becoming increasingly relevant and topical, in which patients are directly involved in a frantic struggle for their freedoms and the doctor who assists them.

An example of this is everything related to informed consent, death with dignity, advance directives, refusal of treatment ... issues that were not taken into account or at least not considered as a priority by our society until a few years ago. Thus, Law 26529 adequately addresses these patient situations.

In its Article 1, it decides on the scope of its application: The exercise of the rights of the patient, in terms of autonomy of will, information and clinical documentation, is governed by the present law. So this legislation is not confrontational with health professionals Rather, they help him in his task. On the other hand, knowing the law makes it more difficult to fall into non-compliance.

154- What is the much written about medical paternalism?

I dare say that the issue of paternalism is a mistake, which was generated from a desk with little knowledge of what a doctor talks about with his patient in very difficult times. From the point of view of health, every thought is valid, but in the face of suffering and in the proximity of the final journey, the doctor's shoulder is the refuge that conveys comfort in the face of pain and death, even if there are no witnesses to what is being said.

From a desk this is not known.

It is striking that profound legal scholars write that doctors treated and treat patients as incapable, that they disregard the projects of each person, that they replace the patient's judgement with that of the doctor, that they reject the patient's wishes, that they deny self-determination. Other writers, emulating a game of chess, say that paternalism has a variant called sacerdotalism, which transforms the physician into the patient's guardian, deciding in his judgement what is best for the patient.

That the patient's wishes are substituted for those of the doctor because he distrusts the doctor's judgement. Paternalism is defined as a mixture of beneficence plus power and that historically this is the idea of this relationship held by most of the law writers who have dealt with this subject. There is no record of anything that was written about it, it is a misconception of writers repeating what someone else wrote.

The patient was never left uninformed, nor did the doctor refuse to accept the patient's wishes, nor is it to be believed symbolically that patients were taken to the operating theatre in chains.

Paternalism, or authoritarianism as someone wrote, is confused with affection, pity and being there for the end. While some men of law discuss transcendent issues such as the importance of procedural law..., the doctor has his shoulder soaked with tears.
This is a totally false and artful imputation of doctors throughout history. As it seems little, some speak of discrimination suffered by the poor,
those who are weak or vulnerable, marginalised or excluded from social life, to those who are ...in all areas of medicine.

So, for the writers of such irresponsibility, the doctors in any sphere of care then discriminate against more tan 20,000,000 inhabitants in Argentina, with just over half of the population being poor and with countless marginalised people.Doctors and other health professionals also have major flaws and imperfections, but they are not exactly those linked to paternalism.

Exceptions exist in every system.

155- What are the most salient concepts of the law?

1-Informed consent. 2-Advance directives
Art.11-Any capable person of legal age may make advance health directives and may consent to or refuse certain medical, preventive or palliative treatments and decisions concerning his or her health.

The directives must be accepted by the attending physician, except for those involving euthanasia, which shall be considered non-existent.

3- The clinical history.

In its art.12 it defines it and its scope

4-Article 22 defines both national and local enforcement authority

It also refers to the right to dignified and respectful treatment, privacy and confidentiality, with emphasis on the autonomy of will and the right to inter-consultation.

156- What is the Difference between Act of God and Force Majeure?

The first refers to the hypothesis of unforeseeability and the second to inevitability. The fortuitous event eliminates the possibility of imputability. Force majeure is a matter directly of liability when it is based on fault.

BY WAY OF CONCLUSION

We can begin this chapter with some of the questions that our readers at will at some point help us to decipher. How can a society with such an excellent medical standard and such a law-abiding and tradition-bound population as the United States have a record number of lawsuits against the medical profession and its health care institutions? The same could be said of France, Italy, Spain. Germany..., where they have long experience in this type of trial. Wasn't it the French who first talked about the medical contract in 1936?

Or are we still not discussing Demogue's theory?

Can we say the same for societies with undisputed historical traditions such as those of most of the East, if they have the same uncontrolled cravings against their doctors? How can it be explained that societies such as those mentioned still have the audacity to attack those who have prolonged their healthy lifespan, ostensibly improved their level of health, changed their diseased organs and, in short, improved their quality of life and prolonged their years of existence? Do we have bad doctors in Argentina and South America? Do low-income patients have access to decent medical care at Argentina and South America? In relation to trials, do the doctors who are accused or the conditions under which they exercise their profession? To the question, if we have bad doctors in Argentina, we can say, without shame, that several generations had and have direct influence of great unequalled masters in our continent. Today's doctors have indeed inherited a distinguished lineage that in one way or another insensibly influences their training up to the present day. I will only name the doctors who come to mind and who are nothing more than the following
more than a part of the forefathers of the 20th century physician and part of the a large number of them are far from my memory and to whom I ask apologies. Let's see whose descendants left traces that are passed down through time almost without us realising it, or at least provided a solid base for other generations to build on and imbibe their knowledge. Let's think of a group of doctors in a disorganised way and who are only some of whom I remember their names. Finochietto, Benain, Agote, **Milstein**, Chacon, Favaloro, **Houssay,** Fustinoni, E.Mazzei, Parodi, Palmaz, Malbran, Mirizzi, I.Goñi Moreno, **Leloir,** H.Faraoni, G.Aranes, I.Bluske, E.Testa... The descendants or those who received technical and human influence from these great men of medicine cannot be bad doctors and although some are not aware of it, they are descendants of these thoroughbreds. They influenced Argentine and American medicine and their preaching is still valid today. However, we see how the merit is eclipsed by any mistakes. This does not mean that medical malpractice does not exist, regardless of the fact that at some point doctors themselves, patients and the entire legal environment should think about the surnames of these medical heroes and find out what their contribution was in the training of generations of doctors. Physicians must constantly remember these men alongside those who dispose of medical legal matters, for they must honour them by their actions. Doctors do not explain well their origin to judges, nor do judges teach and explain the legacy they received from so many legal geniuses, and how they can judge without being doctors. I am almost certain that when reading these untidy lines few are those who Who are they, you may ask?Doctors will also not be able to judge judges lightly on their sentences, as its pedigree begins in antiquity. The Code of Hammurabi existed 1750 years B.C. . The idea

of law was formed when medical knowledge was still in its infancy. Argentine law is, to some extent, underpinned by Argentine law. Roman and its history is one of high birth and distinction.Justinian, Cicero, Grotius, Coke, Kelsen, Beccaria, Gaius, Ulpian, Sassoferrato, Modestinus, Papinianus, Savigny, Ihering, Benthan... Without forgetting more recent ones such as Bustamante Alsina, Bueres, Mosset Iturraspe, Yungano, Lorenzetti, Piedecasas and many more that the limited memory of evocation does not remember them and to whom I apologise. Chiovenda, Atienza, Mazeaud, Enterria ...among so many others, come surprisingly to my memory. This long and tedious list should be a cause for reflection which, although utopian and out of time, would contribute to a better understanding between doctors and judges.

When a medical malpractice file arrives at a judge's chambers, he cannot suspect a priori that he is negligent or something else, as the statement of claim says, he must become even more immersed in the medical problem, thinking that behind the file lies an inheritance of such masters. On the other hand, doctors may or may not agree with a judge's judgement, but it must be respected to the utmost, considering that they are the almost direct heirs of the great founders of the law who surely inspire their judgements.

In any case, doctors and judges are in the middle of a problem that apparently does not seem to exist, but as soon as we go deeper, we will see how they play into the issue of defensive medicine, which, as we studied in the previous chapter, carries a significant percentage of GDP. They are two systems that are central to the balance of society, but they work in silos.

The fearful doctor defends himself or thinks he is defending himself with defensive medicine and the judge applies the Code to the letter, but the lawsuits continue to mount and there is no limit to the money squandered.It is not lost on us that this issue is not exclusively an Argentinean problem, as it is a global issue, in some cases with more intensity than ours. The long and tedious list is a reminder that they are two actors of singular quality and vital to our society. If doctors hold congresses where they discuss how to deal with issues... and lawyers also do so to see if the obligations... we wonder how is it possible to have so much medical and legal sophistication with so little vocation to sit down together, exchange realities, teach, really know each other's work and responsibility? How can they be insensitive to a loss of millions of dollars in a totally bankrupt country? It is not in any way a question of infringing the patient's rights, but of prevent through knowledge a situation that can be improved. The patient-consumer is no stranger to this problem. People are living longer and paradoxically fearing death more and more, which leads to an increased demand for medical benefits, which many professionals accept. We are less and less able to cope with death and cling to the incredible advances of science as a weapon to cope with pain, suffering and old age. Medical advances would be his lifeline and he seeks out the most sophisticated places of care to satisfy his desire for immortality without thinking that the value of the legitimate right to live longer and with a better quality of life comes at a cost. Perhaps with these thoughts we are not asking too much of today's man? Although the illusions grow in greater proportion than some of the results obtained, so it seems that expectations command the hopes of many patients, and are almost always greater than the results. Complicating this equation is the fact that in any part of the world the health resources are limited and needs are infinite. How is it possible that legislatures in Argentina meet to consider that the issue of black pancakes - small dough with burnt sugar on top - is of legislative and provincial interest and others do so to see if relegation in football can be eliminated and a head of a medical service cannot invite a magistrate to breakfast at the hospital so that everyone knows what the real world around them is? Nor does it degrade a magistrate's office, if he invites the director of the hospital and they exchange ideas as to why there are so many complaints from patients? Jump the conventional fences, communicate, exchange ideas, explain what doctors don't know, show doctors what judges don't know. It is not necessary for bureaucratic organisations on bo h sides to intervene to bring these ideas together, do it informally and while reading these proposals go back to the chapter on Defensive Medicine and read over and over again this topic and analyse new forms of calculation.Pricewaterhouse Coopers Health Researche reported that in the US 2.2 trillion dollars a year is spent on healthcare spending, 1.2 trillion dollars could be considered superfluous, avoidable, so-called wastefull spending. Expenditure that could have been avoided without diminishing the quality of medical care. In the US, physicians who practice defensive medicine in the classic specialities are around 90%.

In Italy 94.5 % of gastroenterologists practice defensive medicine in some way, surgeons and anaesthesiologists account for 83 % of the total. Italians spend well over 1 billion euros annually on defensive medicine alone. In Spain, 69% practice defensive medicine, figures from 2002. In Israel, 60% practice defensive medicine.In England (59%) are tests ordered unnecessarily and referrals are also unfounded to specialists (55%).

The fact that the problem of defensive medicine has a global extension does not mean at all that we cannot reduce our figure and you will see what percentage of the GDP it corresponds to. Other countries will be able to bear these costs, but we in Argentina cannot, although we are reducing it considerably. It is of no use if it is to the detriment of the patients, on the contrary, the decrease The cost of expenditure will be in their favour. We all know that the specific role of judges and doctors is not what we propose, but to contemplate our huge expenses without it meaning better medical care or even concern is sinful.

Today's utopias are tomorrow's truths.

With regard to medical care as simple observers we dare to write that the coverage of the high-cost social works, which is e.g. 80% of a minimum monthly pension per person, as already explained, is slowly but steadily becoming more and more like public medicine.

At lower coverages, the problem is exacerbated. And there are systems where input is compulsive and deficient. It is classic to see in the corridors the replica of the diaspora of the Jewish people or the pilgrimage to the Virgin of Lujan, when we see a patient fighting the bureaucracy with a medical order for authorisation, going unsuccessfully through every window i n his path.

Also in the high-cost social security funds, being seen by a specialist means a wait of 45 to 60 days in the best case scenario. Poverty and unemployment never seen before in Argentina means that the public hospital, which is free (although free is a fallacy, as it is paid for with taxes), has a number of patients that exceeds its capacity for the purposes of proper care, which also leads to a loss of quality, mainly in terms of organisation.

In short, medical quality in our country is overshadowed in the private sector by rising costs and the saturation of patients in the public hospital, without forgetting that there are doctors entangled in the economic networks of those who manage health, where commercialisation is the ultimate goal, and as Agrest says, more importance is given to gold than to bronze. The care of pensioners, with a few honourable exceptions, is not really good, even though it is not free of charge.

All this creates an atmosphere of discontent. As we write these lines, TV (2023) informs us that a group of relatives of a patient have just violently destroyed an important part of the ward facilities of the Mercante hospital in José C Paz, Province of Buenos Aires. Violence against health professionals and their institutions must be taken more seriously as it is on the rise and the question is: What is going on?

High costs mean that the quality of medical care is being lost throughout the world, but in Argentina this tendency is magnified and a very negative factor is added when politics gets mixed up in these issues and professional quality is not sought in the management of public medicine, but rather party loyalty.

Although it would be excellent if officials who inaugurate schools and hospitals with eloquent speeches would send their children to these schools and they would be treated in these hospitals.It is not in our spirit to generalise as not everything is the same. Malpractice exists, there are doctors who profit from a favourable certificate to justify e.g. absence from work, there are law firms that hand out cards at the door of hospitals, there are patients whose only aim is to get money at any price, and there are also judges who cannot explain how they got to such a position.

In every system there are exceptions, although the majority of doctors and judges are undoubtedly honourable, which is why it is not difficult for both to understand each other in this problem that we can call the HUNTING OF THE DOCTOR and its consequences.

However, with the exceptions that we reiterate, the patient should perhaps be the object of greater care. The approach is complex, as in our society judges seem to be on a higher rung than doctors and descending is always more complicated.

Perhaps doctors should take the initiative, which is not yet in sight, as we see countless medical congresses without invited judges. We know of exceptions.

They should not be partners or accomplices, but simply have a deep understanding of both responsibilities to an increasingly demanding society.

This claim is supported by a few lines from a couple of judgments that transcribed and which we do not share. The corresponding care of a birth cannot be placed in the category of interventions of doubtful outcome, as it would be creating risks **where there usually are none........**

CNCiv..Sala C ,28-10-86.JA 1987-IV-364 In the situation of maternity hospitals, it is clear that in principle there is an obligation of result, since a normal birth cannot generate risks that cannot be foreseen.......

Cám.Civ.y Com. Morón.Sala II 22-6-88, Juris 87-95 Although these proposals, if they are not conceptually accepted as we propose, then it may be that the problem may be the steps that separate one corporation from another. Mosset Iturraspe in Responsabilidad Civil del Médico, tells us:

We cannot resist the comparison between the doctor and the judge. Both professions can be performed in a pedestrian way or in an almost sacred way.

On the one hand, the doctor or the judge, who do their work to earn their daily bread, only see their job as a way of life and carry it out obeying psychic automatisms, mental habits .... On the other hand, identical characters, judge and doctor, conscious of the dignity and greatness of their work, aware that justice and health are goods of the highest value and that they are the ones in charge of administering them.

Calamandrei, in Eulogy of the Judges, alludes to the question and compares the trembling, the emotion of the old priest at the moment of consecration, with the one that disturbs the judge at the moment of passing sentence, and we would add the doctor, on the occasion of doing something for the health of his fellow man.

Generally, and in response to the question the genesis of the complaints The causes of the judicial system have a multi-causal origin.Continuing with the answers, health care and many social works must have very important improvements as too much of the rope is being pulled, which following the logical order can be broken.... José Núñez Tomás Prosecutor of the High Court of Catalonia: I never thought that the medical profession was so complex and that it had so many repercussions.

Doctors have been clearly judged throughout history: crucifixion was the penalty imposed by Charlemagne on a doctor accused of culpable neglect, and the Fuero Juzgo had the condemnation of handing the doctor over to the The current judicialisation gives the impression that the courts are being used as a measure of force in search of the desired result, although it is a great step forward that society is becoming aware of its rights.

It is not the point of this note to hold up all doctors as innocent victims, as there are professionals who deserve to be prosecuted for various reasons, at least ethically, but they are evidently in the minority, and that there are some, no one doubts.The third factor in discord are the lawyers, about whom one reads issues that Jornet explains very well. As soon as legal fees are reasonable and not exorbitant, perhaps lawyers will stop encouraging people to file unsubstantiated claims.The Rand Corporation, Institute for Civil Justice: The resolution of medical malpractice claims: Modeling the bargaining process.Rep R-27924C/P.M Danzon. Santa Monica,CA, The rand Corporation.1982

Meyerowitz BR, Medical Malpractice and the tort system, JAMA 1990. 263:2180, assessing the situation in the USA, Great Britain and South Africa, concluded that if legal fees were capped at a prudent level, there would be less interest on the part of lawyers in encouraging a potential plaintiff to sue, as it would no longer be a big deal. However, Dazon as well as Sloan argues that the number of lawyers per capita has no significant effect on the frequency of claims or their severity, Danzon is of the opinion that with a 10% increase in new lawyers, malpractice suits increase by 1.2%, stating, "The evidence refutes the hypothesis that lawyer density directly contributes to high claims costs: The evidence refutes the hypothesis that lawyer density directly contributes to high claims costs.

Following Jornet, Sloan argues that the limitation of fees may affect the type of cases chosen by lawyers, but not the severity and frequency of the cases. However, having a good lawyer is essential to win a trial, so much so that some people rightly say: **I didn't win the trial, the**

other side lost it. In summary, the picture in Argentina is bleak, as the medical profession is made up of a minority with an excellent income and a poorly paid majority, together with an unfavourable social mood for all. It is not idle to recall, despite the passing of the years, arguments with which the judges have still underpinned some judgments. They are old, but their concepts are relevant today, both for lawyers and judges, and are in line with earlier chapters. Old failures that should always be present.

Blame

When a man's life and physical integrity are at stake, the slightest imprudence, carelessness or negligence takes on a special dimension which gives it a **singular** gravity. There is no room here for small faults. The proper practice of medicine is incompatible with superficial attitudes. CNCiv. Com.Fed, Chamber I, 8/10/1982. G.J.V v. National Government and others. Rep.LL.1983-655, sum.169.Buenos Aires.

Medical liability

For the purposes of determining medical liability, it is not sufficient to make a generic imputation of errors, negligence or lack of skill on the part of the professionals in charge of the patient's care, but rather a **clear** description is required of the conduct that caused the damage attributed to them, which will be the subject of proof in due course. CNCiv,Sala F,2/9/1983, V.A.M.c/L, J.C and others.Rep.LL, 1984-673 sum.264. The lack of success in the provision of the medical service does not necessarily lead to the obligation to compensate the injured party, since the doctor complies, using the reasonable diligence that can be required of a person who is entrusted with the life of a man or his cure. This is the obligation assumed, since the doctor or surgeon cannot ensure a successful treatment or operation, but only use the appropriate techniques to do so, except in exceptional cases in which liability for a bad result has been accepted. This is because the ultimate success of a treatment or an operation **does not depend entirely** on the practitioner, but is sometimes seen as a result of the use of appropriate techniques. influenced by external factors, such as the surgical risk, the advance of science, or other circumstances that are impossible to control. CNCiv, Sala E, 24/9/1983, R de S, Mc/R and another, ED 119-612, LL, 1986-E 310, JA, 1987-I-259.

BIBLIOGRAPHY

Bueres Alberto.J Responsabilidad Civil de los Médicos, Second Edition, Ed. Hammurabi, Buenos Aires

Barreiro A-La imprudencia punible en la actividad médico-quirúrgica. Ed Tecnos. Madrid.

Cuadernos de Bioética -N 1-Ed AD-HOC-Buenos Aires.

Bello Janeiro Domingo. Responsabilidad civil del médico y Patrimonial de la Administración Sanitaria. Ed ASISA. Madrid 2009.

American Medical Association. Campion F. Grand Rounds on Medical Malpractice Ed AMA.

De Luca M, Galione A, Maccioni S-Responsabilitá Medica.Ed-Gruppo 24 Ore-Third edition-Milan-.

Dodge A-Fitzer S. When Good Doctors Get Sued, Second Edition. Ed Dodge-Associates.USA

Ferrario A, Mariotti P, Serpetti A - Medical Liability

Questioni Processuali.Ed Giuffre-Milan 2010. Milan

Ferreyra Vázquez R-Damages and Damages in the Practice of Medicine. Ed Hammurabi 1992

García Blázquez M-Castillo Calvin J. Ed Comares.Third edition Granada. Spain.

Garay.O.Código de Derecho Médico. Ed AD-HOC 1st Ed.Buenos Aires. Garro de la Colina G. Prevention of Institutional Liability. Private. Ed. ART. La Rioja. Argentina

Iturraspe Mosset J-Piedecasas M-Derecho del Paciente-Ed Rubinzal-. Culzoni 1st edition, Buenos Aires

Jornet J -Malapraxis I ED Ancora, Barcelona, 1991.

Klotz P. Lerreur Medicale. Ed. Maloine Paris 1994

Martínez J M-Pereda Rodríguez -La Responsabilidad Penal del Médico y del Sanitario. Ed Colex 2nd edition -Madrid

Mobilio José. Práctica de Buena Praxis. Ed Nuevo Pensamiento Judicial. San Isidro. Argentina.

Peunneu J. La Responsabilité Médicale, Ed Sirey-Paris.

Pérez de Leal Rosana. Responsabilidad Civil del Médico. Ed Universidad. Buenos Aires.

Represas Trigo F. Reparation of Damages for Medical Malpractice. Ed Hammurabi-Buenos Aires

Sanchez-Caro Abellan F.Derechos del Médico en la Relación Clínica-Ed Comares. Madrid.

Saxton.J-Leaman T.Managed Care Success, Ed Aspen.USA Seecchi E-La Responsabilitá Medica.Ed Giuffre-Milan 2010

Torroni F Aspetti Giuridici From ProfessioneEd Ambrosiana. Milano

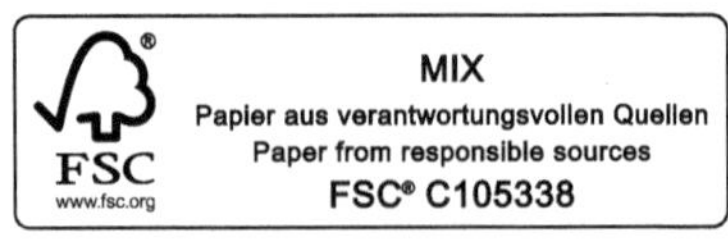

Printed by Books on Demand GmbH, Norderstedt / Germany